CBD Hemp Oil

Ease Pain and Discomfort, Minimize Anxiety and Depression, and Relieve Chronic Illness With Cannabis Oil.

Taylor Rollins

CONTENTS

INTRODUCTION

This book was created to help you better understand CBD Oil and how it can contribute towards improving the health of your loved ones, or even your own. Containing not only an explanation on CBD Oil but also tracing back to the many benefits of its source – the cannabis sativa plant.

Contrary to popular belief, Cannabis Sativa or Marijuana has not always been viewed in such bad light by society. In fact, the plant was highly regarded by many cultures over centuries. In this book, you'll find out exactly how cannabis was used, how it is viewed today, and how it has emerged as a promising super food – especially with the introduction of CBD oil which is a derivation of cannabis sativa.

By the end of this book, you should have a fairly good idea on how to use CBD oil for many ailments and how you can obtain the product given the current laws surrounding marijuana derivatives.

CHAPTER ONE

CBD OIL BASICS

Hearing the word "cannabis" or a derivation of the same word, you would most likely think negative thoughts towards the use of marijuana. This common stereotype attached to the use of CBD Oil or Cannabidiol, often holds a negative belief that Cannabidiol is tantamount to mind-altering drugs.

This is not the case at all.

In this Chapter, you'll find out the distinction between CBD Oil, Hemp Oil, and other derivations from the cannabis plant and why they don't deserve the bad reputation they currently have in society.

Marijuana, Cannabis, and Others

Before we learn about the differences between Hemp Oil and CBD Oil, it's important to first make distinctions between the terminologies that will be used throughout this book. Distinctions should also be made as to what marijuana is, and whether it is synonymous with cannabis and hemp.

Cannabis is synonymous with marijuana, the psychoactive plant. There are two strains of cannabis which are known as Cannabis Sativa and Cannabis Indica. Common belief pronounces that Cannabis Indica has a sedating effect, often used by people to relax at night. Cannabis Sativa on the other hand can be invigorating and promotes creativity in people. Studies have shown however that there's no distinct difference between the effects of these two strains.

So why should there be distinction between the two? While studies have shown that there's no distinct difference between their effects. You will find that most growers believe in the difference between the two in terms of effect. Hence, if you are buying cannabis – you will often be asked if you're looking for the sativa or indica strain. Physically, sativa are tall with narrow leaves. Indica however are shorter in length with broader leaves.

So what is hemp? Hemp is a type of cannabis sativa – making it a favorite for artists or the creative type. Nowadays however, Hemp is produced on an industrial scale and used not just for the production of oil but also for the collection of seeds, fiber, and even CBD.

Hemp Oil vs CBD Oil

Now we touch on the more complicated portion of the discussion. See, all cannabis plants come with hundreds of chemical compounds. Science has advanced far enough that these chemical compounds can be separated, allowing researchers to figure out what compounds produce what kind of effect. For the purposes of this discussion, you'll find that one of the most important chemical compounds is cannabinoids.

Cannabinoids can be further broken down into several types, the most common being THC (Δ9-tetrahydrocannabinol) and CBD (Cannabidiol).

This is where the confusion starts because Cannabinoids sound so similar to Cannabidiol that most people think that Cannabinoids are CBD – but this is NOT the case. Keep in mind that CBD is a type of Cannabinoid.

Why is the distinction important? It's important because THC and CBD have very distinct effects on a person.

- THC – this is the component that makes cannabis psychoactive. It is the chemical compound that produces the high effect as well as relieves pain symptoms, nausea, and producing the feeling of hunger.
- CBD – this is the non-psychoactive compound. It can also help with pain and anxiety as well as other medical ailments – but users of CBD will NOT feel high or intoxicated.

Hence, when we make a distinction between Hemp Oil and CBD Oil – we're primarily talking about the THC or CBD component of each one.

- CBD Oil – is essentially a concentrated liquid purely of CBD or the non-intoxicating part of the cannabis plant. Intake of this oil provides you with ALL the benefits but none of the associated high you'd probably expect from marijuana.
- Hemp Oil – is essentially a concentrated liquid extracted from the Hemp Plant. Hemp Oil may or may not contain THC, depending on how the oil is extracted. Hemp seeds typically do not contain THC and thus, do not have psychoactive effects. However, this is not always the case.

If the hemp oil is removed from any other part of the plant – then some amount of cannabinoids will be included in the oil. We say cannabinoids because the hemp oil may contain both THC and CBD. Typically, it is required for hemp oil manufacturers to label the product, showing buyers exactly how much of the content inside is THC or CBD.

Another important distinction is the plant from which the oil is extracted. Hemp Oil is always extracted from the Hemp plant. However, CBD Oil may be extracted from other types of cannabis sativa. Thus, when we discuss Hemp Oil, we're talking about the plant from where the oil was extracted. When we talk about CDB Oil, we're talking about the chemical compound extracted from any plant belonging to the cannabis sativa family.

Common Misconceptions

So now that distinction has been made when it comes to Hemp Oil and CBD Oil, this book will tackle the common misconceptions or the myths surrounding CBD Oil in general. Here are the facts and fallacies about CBD Oil.

Fact: CBD Oil is NOT psychoactive

CBD Oil, despite being extracted from the cannabis plant, is not psychoactive or does not produce that 'high' effect most people associate with marijuana. CBD is merely a component of marijuana and is not the chemical component which has the intoxicating effect.

Fact: CBD Hemp Oil is Legal in the United States

Notice that we mentioned "CBD Hemp Oil" and not just Hemp Oil. This is because laws regarding CBD Oil use in the United States can be quite confusing with different rules on the national level and the State level. Whether or not you can buy or use CBD Oil in your State depends largely on the State where you reside.

Federal law has classified cannabis as a Schedule 1 drug as per the Controlled Substances Act. This means that the drug has a high potential for abuse. In connection with this, all extracts from the Cannabis plant are also classified as being Schedule 1.

However, what's interesting to note is that industrial hemp is NOT illegal. Hence, if CBD is extracted from the hemp plant – then it becomes completely legal, allowing you to purchase and use it within the United States. Thus, what's legal is CBD Hemp Oil. If the CBD is extracted from any other plant other than Hemp, then it becomes illegal.

Of course, each State has its own law with respect to marijuana with some even allowing recreational use of cannabis. By extension, this also makes CBD Oil legal within the State. Currently, there are 9 states which makes recreational and medical use of marijuana legal. These are: Alaska, California, Colorado, Maine, Massachusetts, Nevada, Oregon, Vermont, Washington, and the District of Columbia.

For the States of Oklahoma, New Mexico, New Jersey, New Hampshire, Georgia, Delaware, Florida, and Connecticut – medical use of marijuana is legal.

Fact: CBD Oil is Different from Medical Marijuana

This has been previously discussed in this book but just to reiterate – CBD is NOT medical marijuana. The two are vastly different with marijuana primarily viewed as illegal or a controlled substance. Component-wise, marijuana still contains THC while CBD Oil is already devoid of the intoxicating component. It must be noted that medical marijuana is primarily used to help with nausea and the management of pain in cancer patients. Both problems are solved through the chemical component THC – which means that medical marijuana must contain the psychoactive element, unlike CBD Oil.

Fact: CBD Oil is Safe for Children

Although further studies need to be made, it has been shown through preliminary research that CBD Oil may be used by children. The oil is primarily used by children suffering from severe epilepsy with promising results – and showing none of the adverse side effects associated with traditional medications. Since there's no THC involved, CBD Oil is actually good for all ages – subject to restrictions on dosage requirements.

Brief History of Cannabis and its Medical Utilization

- **1890s** – hemp production was actually encouraged because it was used for ropes, clothing, and sails.
- **1906** – the Pure Food and Drug Act was enacted which required that any cannabis product be labeled when embedded within over the counter remedies.
- **1900s** – Mexican immigrants originally showed how marijuana can be used recreationally. It was in the 1930s that the fear of marijuana became prevalent. Within the 1930s, the laws concerning marijuana such as the Uniform State Narcotic Act and the Federal Bureau of Narcotics were created.
- **1937** – Marijuana was taxed.
- **1944** - La Guardia Report says that marijuana is not as dangerous as it would appear. This was from the New York Academy of Medicine after an exhaustive research on the plant. Accordingly, marijuana did not induce a person to engage in violence, crimes, or other drug use.
- **1951**- Stricter Sentencing Laws were passed. Specifically, there was the enactment of federal laws (Boggs Act, 1952;

Narcotics Control Act, 1956) which put into place mandatory sentences for the use of marijuana. The first-offense of marijuana possession carried a minimum sentence of 2-10 years with a fine of up to $20,000.

- **1970** – This was the time when marijuana was viewed differently from other drugs, starting the campaign towards its legalization. The National Organization for the Reform of Marijuana Laws (NORML) was founded
- **1986** – Anti-Drug Abuse Act - Mandatory Sentences was passed. This was under the regime of President Reagan which imposed mandatory sentences for drug-related crimes. Together with the Comprehensive Crime Control Act of 1984, federal penalties for marijuana possession and dealing were raised. For example, possession of 100 marijuana plants received the same penalty as 100 grams of heroin. A later amendment to the Anti-Drug Abuse Act established a "three strikes and you're out" policy.
- **1996** – The plant marijuana was eventually legalized in California as treatment for various health problems such as cancer and anxiety.

How Does CBD Oil Work?

The actual workings of CBD Oil is still in progress as the product slowly gains acceptance within the community. The long and short of it is that it helps contribute to the body's maintenance of what is known as homeostasis. This is the body's internal balance and what every organ, cell, and tissue is working towards. If you catch a fever, that's because something is imbalanced inside you and the homeostasis is interrupted. If you lose blood, the homeostasis is obstructed and your body responds by producing more blood cells in order to recreate the balance.

Part of what contributes to the homeostasis of the body is the Enconnabinoid System or ECS. It's a system that reacts exclusively with cannabinoids or CBD. Originally, scientists thought that the ECS system could only be found in rats – but it turns out that it can be found in a variety of species – including humans.

It is the ECS system that interacts with the CBD. Think of CBD as keys and upon entering the body, they work their way towards the ECS and open some unknown portions of the body that contributes to the homeostasis or its balance. This key has been observed to help with numerous ailments, primary of which is its antipsychotic effects, ability to help with pain, mental function, and a person's mood.

Also note that since CBD comes from cannabis, it comes with more or less some of the benefits naturally associated with the plant. Obviously, the element contributed by THC as a hallucinogenic drug does not form part of these benefits and in fact, CBD has the opposite effect.

CHAPTER TWO

CBD OIL BENEFITS

So what exactly can CBD Oil do? Understand that studies are still being conducted with respect to cannabis and its many components, including CBD Oil. So far however, these have been the general consensus of the scientific community with respect to CBD Oil Benefits.

Pain Relief

CBD Oil's ability to relieve pain is one of the primary reasons why it is favored in the scientific community to assist people going through cancer treatments. Marijuana or cannabis from where CBD Oil is derived from, has been historically used to treat pain, tracing all the way back to 2900 BC. When combined with THC, it has been shown to be remarkably effective for reducing inflammation in people with rheumatoid arthritis.

But how exactly does this work? The human body has a system called the endocannabinoid system or ECS which is involved in sleep, immune system functions, appetite, and pain. The body is capable of producing endocannabinoids which comes into contact with cannabinoid receptors. The introduction of CBD in the body does the same thing, binding with the cannabinoid receptors to help reduce inflammation and the consequent nerve pain.

Studies have been done on rats, showing a noticeable decrease in their pain receptors after the introduction of CBD in their system. Under the strength of this study, the oral spray Sativex was introduced in the market which is a combination of THC and CBD. It is currently being used in select countries for the treatment of MS or multiple sclerosis. Accordingly, people who use Sativex have experienced less muscles spasms, better walking control, and less pain within a period of one month. Those with rheumatoid arthritis using Sativex also reported pain relief and better sleep after using the product.

Depression

Depression is a mental health condition that's currently getting much needed attention in the medical community. In animal studies, it has been determined that CBD oil can help alleviate signs of depression in individuals.

Due to the promising results of these tests, most people with depression are naturally drawn to this holistic approach. Currently, depression is being treated with prescribed medications, most of which come with unwanted side effects. Compared to CBD oil, the natural extract appears to be the healthier option, which is why some States are allowing its use for people diagnosed with depression. Note though that the tests are still inconclusive regarding CBD oil and depression.

Anxiety Symptoms

Depression and anxiety are often lumped together with anxiety typically considered a symptom of depression and vice versa. Like depression, anxiety is currently treated with certain drugs which can cause multiple side effects like insomnia, drowsiness, headache, and even sexual dysfunction.

A study – this time involving 24 people diagnosed with social anxiety disorder – showed that people treated with CBD suffer through less anxiety and have less cognitive impairment. More importantly, the oil has been tested on children with anxiety and has been proven to be both effective and safe for the use of minors.

In both depression and anxiety cases, it is theorized that CBD is capable of communicating with the brain's serotonin receptors, allowing for improvement on social behavior and mood.

Cancer Related Symptoms

The primary use for medical marijuana and CBD nowadays is in relation to cancer and cancer treatment. Pain is the most debilitating symptom of cancer which, according to studies, may be treated with the use of CBD.

In a study conducted on 177 people suffering from pain brought about by cancer, the use of CBD combined with THC managed to lower the amount of pain they experienced from the condition. These 177 people were chosen specifically because their pain can no longer be handled by traditional medication – which meant that in their cases CBD with THC provided a more effective solution in comparison to other pain medications.

It must also be noted that one of the effects of cannabis is to reduce vomiting and nausea in people. These problems are often side effects of chemotherapy, thus making CBD combined with THC an excellent solution for people going through chemotherapy. Accordingly, a simple mouth spray of CBD and THC in equal parts can help reduce symptoms of nausea and vomiting significantly better than standard treatments.

Current studies also promote the possibility of CBD in itself being a treatment for cancer. It allegedly has anticancer properties as observed in test-tube studies with concentrated forms of CBD capable of killing breast cancer cells. Of course, these studies are still in the study phase and need to be properly researched and tested before final conclusions can be made.

Heart Health

Some studies today claim that CBD may be helpful to heart health. Although, these studies are still in their infancy stage. More specifically, CBD can help lower high blood pressure which is one of the biggest killers related to the cardiovascular system.

In a study, men were administered 600mg of CBD Oil and were found to have a lowered resting blood pressure compared to the control group. To further test the extent of CBD oil, the same men were made to undergo stress to see if their blood pressure would increase. While there was a slight elevation, said increase of the blood pressure was less than that of the control group.

Acne

While CBD as an acne cure may seem like such a small thing compared to its ability to help with cancer and other problematic health conditions, it must be noted that a large number of the population suffer from this skin disorder. Roughly 9% of the total population have this problem, many of which suffer from severe acne which drastically lowers the quality of their life.

Since CBD has anti-inflammatory properties, it is theorized that CBD oil can help with the complications brought on by acne. If applied correctly, it can also moderate the production of sebum which is an oil produced by the skin which can lead to pimples. Overproduction of sebum tends to block the pores, thereby causing dirt and grime to remain stuck underneath, leading to an irritation or a pimple. With the application of CBD, the amount of sebum produced is not only lowered but any sign of inflammation is quickly tapered down, reducing the instances of a breakout.

Neuroprotective Properties

While this might feel like a reiteration of what has already been mentioned, it bears revealing that CBD Oil may have a positive effect on neurological disorders. This basically means any disorder related to the nervous system – the most common of which are epilepsy, multiple sclerosis, and Parkinson's disease.

With a neurological disorder, patients suffer degenerative functions attacking the brain and the nerves that connect them all over the body. Hence, people with neurological disorders have a hard time moving, swallowing, or gaining control over the movement of their limbs.

There is promising research that CBD has neuroprotective properties in that it can help prevent the onset of symptoms related to neurological diseases. Sativex is an oral spray that is currently being used by multiple sclerosis patients in helping not just with pain but also with their movement problems. This oral spray is a combination of THC and CBD.

Here are some neurological diseases and the benefits they achieved from using CBD Oil:

- Huntington's Disease – helps improve symptoms of the disease through reduced tremors
- Parkinson's Disease – improves their quality of life by reducing tremors and better quality of sleep
- Alzheimer's Disease – it managed to delay and prevent neurodegeneration for patients, allowing to hold on to their cognitive faculties for longer periods of time

Anti-Psychotic Properties

As uncanny as it might sound, studies have shown that CBD may have anti-psychotic effects. Remember that CBD is that part of marijuana that doesn't have intoxicating properties and as it turns out, it might actually do the opposite for people suffering from psychotic disorders. A study used CBD oil on people suffering from schizophrenia and found that it can help manage the symptoms.

Overcoming Substance Abuse

CBD Oil is allegedly capable of modifying the circuits of the brain so as to stamp out drug-seeking behavior. When taken as is, the oil can reduce dependence on certain addictive drugs such as heroin and morphine. However, this study has only been conducted on rats so there's still countless tests and research needed to learn about the role of CBD oil in substance abuse.

Anti-Tumor

As previously mentioned, it's been found that CBD is capable of attacking cancer cells. In animals, CBD has been used to prevent breast, brain, colon, lung, and prostate cancer cells from multiplying. Studies on humans have not yet been forthcoming so there's still much that needs to be done about the product.

Preventing Diabetes

Conducted on diabetic mice, studies show that the introduction of CBD as treatment can help reduce the instances of a diabetic attack by 56%.

CHAPTER THREE

CBD OIL SIDE EFFECTS

After talking about CBD Oil benefits in the last Chapter, it's time to talk about the side effects associated with the liquid. While there's no question that CBD Oil has its good side, the fact is that there are still risks associated with its intake.

Dosage Issues

CBD Overdose is a distinct possibility, especially if you're taking it without the guidance of a licensed physician. The problem with CBD oil use is that people think few drops of oil is not enough in order to obtain the results they want.

What you have to remember however that CBD Oil is much like essential oils in that they are as pure and as concentrated as possible. Hence, even a few small drops would be able to produce excellent results. Later on in this book, we'll talk about how to use CBD oil and the proper dosage to be used depending on the person.

Extraction Issues

Perhaps the most prevalent risk associated with CBD Oil is the fact that you can never really tell how the oil is extracted. National regulations require that CBD Oil is extracted in a specific way and that the components of the oil must be properly shown on the label. Unfortunately, this may not always be the case, making it crucial for buyers to thoroughly scrutinize products before making their purchases. The maxim caveat emptor plays a big role here as the CBD Oil industry may not be as regulated as one would hope. If you think the CBD Oil product is too cheap, then chances are there are the product is inferior and may interfere with any results you wish to achieve.

Complications with Other Medications

It must also be noted that despite being 100% natural, CBD oil may interact negatively with other medications, specifically those used with epilepsy. Studies have shown that when taken together with certain medications, CBD actually worsens the symptoms of epilepsy instead of providing relief. Thus, you'd want to make sure that you're not worsening the condition by taking CBD Oil. If you really want to include CBD Oil in your treatment, ask your primary physician first about any possible interactions. Note that while some doctors today are open to the use of CBD oil, others may not be as open to the idea.

CHAPTER FOUR

WHERE TO BUY AND WHAT TO LOOK FOR

Buying CBD Oil – whether through a store or through the internet. As mentioned, the buyer is encouraged to be aware of the different brands available, the regulations governing the production of CBD Oil, as well as the brands that are worth buying and proven among other consumers. To reiterate – cheap is not always better. Quality is what you should be after and if that means buying the slightly more expensive CBD Oil, then so be it.

In this Chapter, we'll talk about the different products available in the market today and what you should look for when buying and using CBD.

What Type of Products Are Available?

This will be discussed more extensively in a later Chapter but for purposes of this discussion, you should know that there are capsules, creams, oils, tinctures, and e-liquids made from CBD Hemp Oil. While you have the freedom of buying any of those, this Chapter will focus primarily on CBD Hemp Oil.

Why Choose CBD Oil?

While you can get CBD Oil capsules and gels, the use of the tincture or liquid version is usually preferable if you're getting CBD oil for a host of reasons.

For example, if you want to try out CBD oil specifically to help with Type 1 Diabetes, then it makes sense to get gels or capsules so you'll be more accurate with the dosage. However, if you want CBD oil for a more all-around cure such as when you have headaches, acne, psoriasis, anxiety, and the like – all at the same time – then you'll want to obtain CBD Oil. This is because of all the types available today – CBD Oil is the most flexible in terms of use, application, and dosage. While capsules typically come in 400mg, 500mg, or 600mg, you can go as low as 100mg with CBD oil and control your dosage.

If you're new and unsure of how much you should be getting, then the CBD oil will allow you to properly figure out your optimum dosage.

Choosing CBD Oil – Tips to Remember

Find Out Your Current Legal Status

This is important if you're buying online because the product you choose to buy may not be approved within your country or State. Remember that while CBD oil is legal in many countries. There's a restriction as to how much THC content must be included. Hence, you'll have to know how much THC content is permissible in your current location. Once you know your limits, you can start your search.

Know Where the Hemp or Main Plant is Grown

The CBD oil is extracted from cannabis and you'll need to know where this cannabis plant was cultivated. Why? Marijuana or cannabis plants are known as hyper-accumulators. This makes them very good in absorbing any sort of mineral or chemical within the soil. In fact, cannabis plants are often used to help rid the soil of toxins because they can take those toxins and incorporate them in their own parts. Simply put, if the cannabis is grown in bad soil, then the extracted CBD oil will contain traces of those bad chemicals.

So how do you know that the CBD oil is grown well? Look for labels indicating that the hemp is grown in the United States. The US currently has a regulating system imposed by the department of agriculture to make sure that the quality of hemp grown is maintained. Ideally, this information is stated in the manufacturer's website.

Look at THC Content

As already mentioned, you have to know how high you can go with respect to THC. Since THC is the intoxicating property associated with cannabis, States can be quite strict when imposing this limitation. This limit varies from one State to the next, but the usual amount is roughly 0.3 percent so try not to go beyond that limit. Note though that the amount of THC in the CBD Oil is not indicative of quality. Even if the THC content is just 0.1%, the CBD oil in itself may be poorly drawn and thus, will not provide you with the results you want.

Opt for Whole Plant Extracts

This refers to the portion of the plant from where the CBD was extracted. Whole plant extracts mean exactly that – that every part of the cannabis plant was utilized in order to get the CBD oil.

This is crucial in the overall scheme of thing because getting CBD from all parts means that the extract can include other compounds that work well with CBD. For example, it can contain flavonoids, terpenes, and other cannabinoids that help produce the positive effect you want – all that's missing is the THC.

Note that some brands use the term "Full Spectrum" instead of whole plant which means basically the same thing. This is an option though and if you can't find CBD oils that are derived from the whole plant, then the alternative will work just as well for the purposes stated.

Choose Organic

Try to opt for organic as possible when buying CBD Hemp Oil products. Remember that cannabis is a hyper accumulator so any pesticides or chemicals sprayed on them are likely to be absorbed by the plant.

An organically grown product means that you'll be receiving CBD oil in its purest form – with no added harmful chemicals. Today, there are several places that produce organically grown CBD oil which include Kentucky and Colorado.

Don't Focus on the Price

This is the case of things being too good to be true. Remember that you'll be putting the CBD oil into your body – which means that it has to be perfectly made with the promised benefits and none of the negative side effects. It stands to reason that a quality product will have a price to match – so try not to be too stingy with the cost. Look for a middle ground when it comes to pricing and don't be sold into the cheapest options available in the market. In fact, it's usually better to go by brand for your first purchase.

Third Party Verification

Third party lab results should be made available to buyers in order to create transparency and trustworthiness between the brand and its consumers. A third party laboratory will help make sure that the

CBD oil meets the general guidelines set up by the State for the overall health and wellbeing of its users. Look at the seller's website – they should be able to provide verification by a third party laboratory which is also named therein. Don't be lazy with your research and dig a little deeper. Google the name of the laboratory mentioned and check to see if the laboratory in itself has a good reputation in the industry. Remember this is your health.

Check the Third Party Laboratory

As mentioned, you should check the laboratory which performed the verification. A third party laboratory has no financial interest in the CBD oil and thus is not inclined to lie for the benefit of the CBD brand. Again, the laboratory itself must have a good reputation.

The first thing you should look for is the certification of the laboratory which should be ISO-17025 certified. This is the gold standard and are being used by top medicinal products in the market today. Examples of these laboratories include Steep Hill, SC Global, Erofins, and ProVerdo.

Second, check to see how the laboratory does the assessment. They shouldn't just be looking at the concentration of CBD and THC levels but also testing for possible contaminants such as residual solvents, heavy metals, pesticides, herbicides, micro biologics, and phytocannabinoid spectrum. A good source of help when comparing third party laboratories is the Anavii Market.

Avoid Those with Health Claims

As weird as this may sound, it's usually not a good idea to buy CBD oil with labels that promote certain health benefits or have health claims. Yes, this book is primarily premised on the idea that

CBD oil has multiple health benefits – but this limitation has its basis on law.

The Food and Drug Administration prohibits the making of any health claim on CBD products – primarily because there's still a need to fully study the compound. Without an exhaustive study on CBD and verification from the medical community, all health claims are premature and should not be used as a basis for marketing the product. If the product claims to cure cancer or stop pain, then there's potentially something wrong with it and you'll have to look for a different brand.

Stay as Pure as Possible

The great thing about CBD oil is that it stays as true to the cannabis plant as possible. This means that there's rarely any unnecessary ingredients added into the product which can significantly alter how it works. A good example here is e-liquid CBD which is used with a vaporizer. Later on in this book, you'll find that an e-liquid CBD can actually be used for smoking – but that's only one of the options for using CBD products to help you quit smoking. While it is possible, it's generally discouraged. This is because CBD e-liquid comes with thinning agents which are added to the compound so that they'll work better with the vaporizer.

The rule is that if you can use CBD oil as is for the purpose you want, then you should stick to it instead of using other CBD infused products. Note that flavorings added to CBD are also best avoided.

Check the Extraction Method

This is where things can get a bit technical but what you simply need to know is that there are several ways that CBD oil can be separated from THC and the plant in general. This is one of the primary factors affecting the price of the product. With less sophisticated extraction methods, you'll find that the chemicals you don't want are still embedded within the CBD oil. It's cheaper but it's also more of a risk to your health.

The extraction process you're looking for is through the use of carbon dioxide or Supercritical CO2 Extraction. What happens is that carbon dioxide is exposed to high pressure, which isolates the CBD oil while at the same time maintaining and preserving the purity of the extract. Due to the sophistication and precision of the extraction process, expect to shell out a bit more for the product. However, it is definitely worth it and highly recommended.

Other methods include the use of coconut oil or CBD oil. Since these substances are not harmful per se, they're also good methods for extraction, but not in the same level as the use of carbon dioxide.

The good news is that most CBD manufacturers are upfront about their extraction method. Hence, you won't have to dig deep in order to get the answers you want. Just make a point of verifying the information they give you through further research.

Check the Concentration

The concentration refers to how much mg of CBD oil is contained per ml of the product. You'll typically find this on the label and knowing this information gives you a fairly good idea on how to estimate dosage. However, the concentration should also tell you if you're getting your money's worth.

For example, if the concentration is just 100mg per serving – then you're getting a pretty bad deal if the price is practically the same as one with a 3000mg per serving. Do the math at this point, taking into account how much oil you'll be using during the day. The only good thing about small concentration CBD oil is that you'll have more control over the amount you take in because you can increase or decrease by smaller increments.

CHAPTER FIVE

LEGALITIES OF BUYING AND USING CBD OIL

We've already touched upon the legality of marijuana and in connection with it, CBD Oil, with respect to the United States. However, you'll find that with the world wide impact of CBD Oil in the medical community, various regulations are also being established by different countries.

It's important to make a distinction between buying, selling, and using CBD with respect to different countries. For purposes of this book, we'll discuss the legal status of CBD oil in the United States and the United Kingdom.

First thing first, keep in mind that this book discusses CBD Oil in particular. While there are currently numerous products that have been infused with CBD – such as CBD chocolates – the subject of their legality will not be discussed in this Chapter.

United States

The general consensus is that the United States has made CBD Oil legal. This means that you can buy CBD Oil everywhere within the United States – including online stores. However, there are still exceptions to this, primarily on the source or the derivation of

CBD. As previously mentioned, CBD can be extracted from the cannabis sativa plant – but which type of cannabis sativa? If the CBD is extracted from Hemp, then it is considered legal. However, if it is extracted from marijuana, then the CBD is considered illegal.

Therefore, you'll have to be careful about the CBD Oil derivation. A distinction is made because Hemp contains zero or very low levels of THC – the intoxicating chemical compound in cannabis sativa. On the other hand, marijuana contains a higher concentration of THC which means that it would be hard to extract CBD without a little bit of THC being included in the resulting oil.

So if you're going to buy CBD Oil, you'll have to take a good look at where you live in the United States. If you live in any of the following States, then you're in luck! CBD Oil may be bought for medicinal and recreational use. We're talking about CBD oil that's derived from both Hemp and Marijuana here. Note though that there's still a limit as to how much you can have on your person when it comes to marijuana but for the most part, marijuana and hemp have been decriminalized in these States:

- Alaska
- California
- Colorado
- Maine
- Massachusetts
- Nevada
- Oregon
- Washington

If you'll notice, those States decriminalized marijuana and hemp in their plant form and by extension, all its derivatives – including CBD Oil.

But what if you only want to buy CBD Oil and not the actual plant? If you live in any of these 29 States, then you can buy CBD Oil – subject to the presence of a prescription from a doctor. Hence, these 29 States allow the use of CBD oil from hemp or marijuana, provided it is for medical purposes:

- Alaska
- Arizona
- Arkansas
- California
- Colorado
- Connecticut
- Delaware
- Florida
- Hawaii
- Illinois
- Maine
- Maryland
- Massachusetts
- Michigan
- Minnesota
- Montana
- Nevada
- New Hampshire
- New Jersey
- New Mexico
- New York
- North Dakota
- Ohio
- Oregon
- Pennsylvania
- Rhode Island

- Vermont
- Washington
- West Virginia
- Guam
- Puerto Rico

It must be noted that since CBD Oil in these states can be derived from either hemp or marijuana, there's a specific limit as to how much THC is contained in the CBD Oil. Limits range between 0.3% to 8% so make sure that your CBD Oil of choice falls within the range required by your State.

Unfortunately, some States still view cannabis and cannabis-derived products to be bad and thus, have not passed legislation making them legal for use, medical or otherwise. These four States currently view marijuana as illegal:

- Idaho
- Kansas
- Nebraska
- South Dakota

The laws are currently vague with respect to CBD so you might find some people who use CBD oil for medical purposes living in these States. New developments are ongoing as of this writing which should change the way these States view CBD Oil.

Europe and the United Kingdom

Medical use of cannabis is legal in several countries found in Europe and as an extension of which, makes CBD Oil equally legal. These countries are:

- Austria
- Belgium
- Denmark

- Netherlands
- Romania
- Spain
- Italy

Hemp cultivation is also legal, which makes it easy to obtain hemp-derived CBD Oil provided that the THC level is no more than 0.2 percent. Note though that CBD taken from the cannabis plant is still illegal as per the Misuse of Drugs Act of 1971, which can be quite confusing for most.

Switzerland

Switzerland's approach to the cannabis issue is tackled through the Swiss Narcotic Act which makes THC illegal but CBD Oil legal. If the CBD Oil contains less than 1% of THC, then it can be produced, sold, and purchased within the country.

Canada

Canada perhaps has one of the most forward-thinking legislations when it comes to cannabis use. Cannabis has been made legal for all purposes – including medicinal use. The execution of the law allowing this is still in the works though so pending actual passage, cannabis is currently being regulated from medicinal purposes only. However, CBD Oil is easily obtained by users with no actual restriction with respect to THC levels.

CHAPTER SIX

HOW TO CONSUME CBD OIL AND DOSAGES

While there are tons of articles and studies regarding the benefits of CBD oil, very few actually talk about the proper use of the product. Since questions as to legality as still up in the air, not much study has been made on how it can actually be incorporated for medical purposes. Right now, there are suggestions but for the most part – individuals are told to observe their intake and increase or decrease the amount, depending on the side effects achieved. In this Chapter, we'll try to narrow down CBD Oil dosage and how it can be used for common health problems like headaches, acne, nausea, inflammation, and others.

Types of CBD Oil Products in the Market

First, you should know that CBD Oil comes in various forms today, depending on which one you find most useful. There's really only 4 though and your purchase would depend on how it will be used:

- CBD Oil Extract – this is perhaps what you picture when you think CBD Oil. The oil typically comes in a small bottle with a droplet at the top. The content is pure liquid and is typically added to other concoctions to get the results you want. For example, it's generally added to moisturizers to help fight acne.

- CBD Soft Gel – if you're taking CBD for medical purposes like to help with muscle pain or to help control certain neurological problems, the soft gel version is perhaps the best. Studies on CBD typically involve the use of 600mg of oil taken internally but many soft gels contain less than that. If you're going to use CBD soft gel, you should check the label and follow the recommended dosage on the product.
- CBD Capsule – this is virtually the same as soft gel.
- CBD Vape Oil – this version of the CBD product is limited for the use of people who want to quit smoking. Instead of cigarettes, you use CBD Vape Oil for your vaporizer to reduce the signs and symptoms of nicotine withdrawal.

How Much Should You Use?

This is really the million-dollar question. If your doctor prescribed the use of CBD Oil, then it stands to reason that he'll also give a suggestion on proper dosage. If not however, you are left to figure out how much you should take and how often. The tricky part here is that some doctors have no idea on what the proper dosage actually is. This is because there's really no standard regulation on how much can and must be taken in order to address a specific health problem.

There is NO recommended dietary allowance for CBD – but that doesn't mean you can take as many as you wish. The rule of thumb is to take one drop of CBD Oil per day, but this is actually dependent on a number of factors such as what you're trying to cure, how much you weigh, the concentration of CBD, etc.

Here's a guide on how to figure out the proper dosage for you.

Step 1: Use Your Weight as Basis

More body mass means more CBD dosage in order to make sure that every part of you gets the benefit of the oil. The rule of this is 1mg to 6mg of CBD for every 10 pounds. The amount you take is also dependent on the level of pain you currently have.

The general rule is to start at the low end of the spectrum and just gradually increase the amount if the pain is still present. If your doctor has prescribed the dosage you take, then you'll obviously have to follow that. However, if you're doing this at your own initiative, then you'll have to be very careful with the dosage. Check out this website to help you properly figure out how much dosage you should be getting: honestmarijuana.com/dosage-calculator.

It is strongly recommended that you determine your dosage personally and not use someone else as a basis. For example, you have a friend using CBD Oil too and since you're the same weight, you figured you'll use the same dosage. Remember that you're computing dosage not just on the basis of weight but also with respect to your pain tolerance and level of pain experienced. Plus, there's also the fact that body chemistry is different from one person to another.

Traditional medicines have a standard weight to dosage ratio because they've undergone extensive research and thus have a solid background for the suggestions. Unfortunately, this is not the case for CBD – which means that you'll have to be more careful. This is not to say that CBD oil is dangerous per se but simply a technique to make sure you're not taking in more than you're supposed to.

Step 2: Consult Your Physician

This should really be in Step 1, but if you find yourself having negative effects, stop the CBD oil use immediately and consult with your physician. Ideally though, you should consult your physician beforehand – especially if you're taking medications along with CBD oil.

For example, you may be using medication for diabetes or high blood pressure. The possibility of interaction between these two drugs can definitely have an impact of how the CBD affects your body. Do your research, taking into account the specific medication you're using and contrasting them with the use of CBD oil.

Fortunately, the internet is helpful enough that you can get decent information online about what it would be like if you take CBD oil and certain drugs at the same time. Note though that online information is usually superficial so you'd want to dig a little deeper with research. Your doctor would be the one capable of giving you the best information about the matter.

Step 3: Try Not to Introduce Anything New to Your Body

Try not to do anything new or extreme in the meantime. This means not doing anything that will probably affect how the CBD oil will change your body. This means getting rid of any medications that you can live without and were not prescribed to you. For example, if you're taking certain vitamins or plan to start taking them, you might want to skip that and just concentrate on using CBD oil for now. Steer clear of any cleanses or any extreme diets and just keep your day to day life on the regular until you've properly assessed what CBD oil can do to your overall health and mood.

Step 4: Observe Yourself Over the Next Days

Obviously, you'll have to be a little more self-aware during the following days, trying to figure out how the CBD oil is changing your body. Do you feel better about yourself? Is your mood getting better? Is your acne fading away? These are things you'll have to greatly consider during the next few days or weeks.

There's no specific amount of time to follow before you can get results. It's alleged that CBD oil reacts quickly which means that you should be able to observe results within the day after taking the oil. Of course, this would still depend on the kind of use you're getting from the product. For example, if you're using it to control acne, then 3 weeks should be the minimum amount of time for observation to find out if the product is actually working for you.

Getting Specific with Dosage

Here's a little problem you might have to deal with when using CBD Oil – how much mg is there in a single drop? While the CBD Oil bottle tells you the quantity inside the bottle, there's no telling how much you get with each drop.

There are several ways you can work with this starting with conversion of ml to mg. You can use a syringe to take out the CBD oil and then convert the resulting ml to mg. One refers to volume while the other refers to mass – which makes the conversion quite complicated, but this should at least give you some approximation on the product. The same technique can work with CBD oil vape liquid which is consumed through smoking – which makes the estimation of dosage a bit more difficult.

With CBD tincture, the rule of thumb is to use one drop administered orally, but how much mg can you get per drop? There's actually a formula for this so you'll have to be patient as it's explained. A dropper contains around 1ML of liquid. Find out how much ml the CBD oil bottle you have and then use this formula:

Total number of CBD oil in bottle / number of ml in bottle = mgs of CBD per dropper or per ml

Of course, you can also use the internet to easily make the conversion through online calculators. Accuracy is not 100% but this should at least give you a decent starting point to figure out how much you actually need. The same technique applies for when using e-liquid CBD for vaping. Pay close attention to how much you're putting in the tank of your CBD and how long it takes you to consume the whole tank.

At the end of the day however, you'll find that there's one surefire way of getting results: by using CBD oil capsules or soft gels. With this method, you should be able to get the exact dosage you need without any problems.

In the next chapter, we'll talk about how to actually use CBD oil for various ailments.

CHAPTER SEVEN

HEALTH BENEFITS AND HOW TO PROGRESS WITH CBD OIL

So how do you start using CBD Oil? Using CBD oil depends largely on the kind of health problem you want to deal with. Here are some of the most common ailments solved by CBD oil and how you're supposed to use the product to get the results.

Relieve Pain and Inflammation

If you're going to use CBD oil for back pain, inflammation, or any kind of pain – you have several options available. Oddly enough, applying the oil directly to your back is not one of those options as topical application will not give you the result you want. There's low permeability to CBD oil – which basically means that it won't be able to go deep when passing through the pores of the skin. So what do you do instead?

The best way is through oral intake. Place one drop of CBD oil in the back of your tongue and allow it to stay there for 30 to 60 seconds. Swallow afterwards and you should be able to feel some relief within the hour. If you prefer, you can also get CBD gel capsules with a higher concentration of CBD oil. Take them as needed whenever you experience back pain.

Headaches and Migraine

Headaches and migraines are two very different kettles of fish. Migraines go beyond the typical pain level and can last from 4 to 72 hours. Painkillers are often capable of helping with both headaches and migraines, but recent studies took to the use of CBD with some success for alleviating the problem, particularly migraines.

Now, there are several recommended ways to administer CBD oil for headaches. First is by taking a dropper and placing a drop of CBD oil under your tongue. Wait for 60 seconds before swallowing, allowing the oil to thoroughly seep through your body.

- You also have the option of smoking CBD oil through the help of a vaporizer and e-liquid CBD oil. This is hailed as the better option because smoking actually delivers the CBD compounds faster to your body, which means that you'll get better results. If you're experiencing severe pain, vaping is also the better option overall.
- Of course, if you're not familiar with vaping, then oral CBD oil will work just as well. It must be noted that between oral and smoking, the oral ingestion of CBD oil is actually the safer of the two and less likely to cause side effects. While there's no specific guideline to follow for CBD dosages for migraines, you can start with 2.0 or 2.5 mg per day. That means you can possibly use 2 drops of CBD oil under your tongue throughout the day.
- You can also try applying the CBD oil directly to the portions of your head where the pain is localized.

However, this may not work as well as intake through inhalation or through oral treatment.

- Another notable method of using CBD oil for migraines is through a nebulizer. That's right – you put CBD oil in a nebulizer and inhale the smoke coming out of the device. A nebulizer is the same device you use for taking asthma medication, but it can also be used for cannabis oil, thereby allowing the oil to enter your bloodstream faster. But what about diffusing it using a typical diffuser? That's usually not a good idea.

Help with Acne and Psoriasis

When using CBD oil for your skin, the typical application is usually topical. This means applying the CBD product directly to your face in order to control the growth of pimples and the spread of psoriasis. If you can purchase CBD cream in your current location, then you'll find that this is the better option for acne and psoriasis. If you're using CBD oil in bottled products however, you'll have to be a little more creative. You can do any of the following:

- Put one or two drops onto your daily moisturizer and blend the oil completely on the cream. Apply this to your face as usual. CBD oil comes with antibacterial properties which should discourage irritation resulting to breakouts. The same technique works for psoriasis.
- You can also take CBD oil orally using the method described above. Make sure the oil is dropped on the back of your tongue and allow it to spread a little in your mouth for 60 seconds before swallowing.
- You can also apply the oil directly on the skin, specifically on the parts that you want to treat. What you have to remember however is that CBD oil has a low permeability.

This means that while the oil can pass through the pores, you'll need a generous amount in order to get the results you want. If you're using CBD oil as is – try to be as generous as possible in the application.

- Lastly, you can take in CBD oil through capsules or soft gels. Through this intake, you should be able to benefit all over and not just with acne or psoriasis issues.

Cancer Treatment Relief

This is perhaps the most controversial yet one of the most accepted uses for CBD oil. Today, cannabis is actually administered by doctors for their cancer patients in conjunction with other medications, to help with cancer relief. Although the theory that cannabis actually helps prevent cancer is still in doubt, there's no question that CBD can help alleviate the symptoms associated with cancer treatment.

As mentioned, cancer treatment usually involves the use of chemotherapy. Chemotherapy has the effect of causing hair fall, extreme fatigue, and nausea. It hits on the immune system, causing patients to be extremely weakened after each dosage. The use of CBD however helps manage these side effects of treatment, specifically when it comes to the effect of nausea. By extension, it also helps boost the immune system so that patients will have an added boost of energy after the treatment.

It's also proven that CBD oil can help with pain management. People who suffer through cancer-associated pain have been switched to cannabis use after their pain can no longer be managed by traditional medication. The result is astounding as the patients report better pain tolerance.

But how exactly are you supposed to use CBD oil for cancer treatment relief? Usually, it's best to have your doctor suggest and monitor the dosage for this. Most doctors have no problem prescribing CBD oil if the same is not illegal in your current State. Others will go as far as to prescribe medical marijuana so as to give you the full benefits of the plant.

If no prescription is available, you can take CBD Oil orally by placing it under your tongue for 60 seconds before swallowing. Studies show that most doctors use around 400mg to 600mg of CBD oil for cancer-related pain so you can make use of that estimate or better yet, use the calculator given earlier in this book to figure out the dosage you'll need. Capsules or soft gels are also idea if you prefer a simpler way of introducing CBD in your system.

Highly Effective with Seizures and Epilepsy

It's not known exactly how CBD oil helps with seizures and epilepsy – but there's no question that they do. A case study which will be discussed later, has shown that the routine intake of CBD oil not only reduces seizures but also gives patients ample control over the severity of their seizures. This is especially true for people who suffer from seizures that are non-responsive to traditional drugs. If you can get the go signal from your doctor to include CBD oil in your medication, then this should go a long way in helping with the complications of seizures and epilepsy. In the study, the dosage given was 600mg per patient administered over a period of one year.

Type 1 Diabetes

There's a distinct difference between Type I and Type II Diabetes in that Type 1 Diabetes is not at all preventable.

Type 1 Diabetes is characterized by the body's inability to produce insulin. It's a disease wherein your own body mistakes healthy cells as invaders, causing them to attack the cells which produce insulin. This usually occurs early in life and requires treatment through the injection of insulin in the bloodstream on a routine basis.

Type 2 Diabetes on the other hand is the most common today and happens due to lifestyle choices. Obese people have the highest risk of Type 2 Diabetes characterized by the body's inability to recognize the presence of insulin.

So how does CBD Oil help with Type 1 Diabetes? It is alleged that with CBD Oil, the following symptoms of Type 1 Diabetes can be better managed:

- It helps prevent diabetic complications such as the buildup of plaque in the arteries which can also lead to heart issues.
- CBD Oil can also help prevent damage to the cells and nerves. You'll note that diabetes usually causes a person to feel tingling or numbness, which is indicative of problems with the nerves. CBD Oil should help prevent these problems and by extension, remove the possibility of amputations which is often needed by diabetic patients due to nerve damage.
- It also helps with glucose intolerance, which means that sugar won't affect you as badly as it used to. Your body will have better chances of recognizing insulin, which means that your dosage of insulin may be lowered as the CBD oil does its job.

Now the question is – how do you administer CBD oil for Diabetes Type 1? There are several ways available, depending on your personal preference. Here are your choices:

- You can take the CBD gels or capsules in the recommended dosage as provided for in the product's label

- You can also use CBD Oil orally following the instructions already given in this book.

Note though that if you're diagnosed with Type 1 Diabetes, then chances are you're also taking medications to help with the condition. If this is the case, it is absolutely vital that you tell your doctor about your plans to use CBD oil. This will help them properly assess whether an interaction between the two compounds can cause negative side effects to your health. For the most part however, negative interactions is not a problem.

Type 2 Diabetes and CBD

What about Type 2 Diabetes? It is suggested that CBD Oil can work just as well with Type 2 Diabetes. As already mentioned, Type 2 Diabetes typically results from lifestyle choices and occurs gradually as an individual consumes or focuses on eating unhealthy food products.

In comparison to Type 2 Diabetes, Type 1 patients still produce insulin in their body – it's just that their body is not capable of recognizing the insulin. Hence, the treatment is not the introduction of insulin but rather, a way for the body to recognize the compound again.

What can CBD Oil do for people with Type 2 Diabetes? Here are some of the benefits:

- Helps with insulin resistance. This means that your body will have a higher chance of recognizing the insulin levels, allowing for better balance. There's no clear rule as to how CBD manages to do this – but doctors are of the opinion that this relates to CBD's anti-inflammatory properties.
- CBD oil can also help prevent obesity. Remember that obesity is one of the leading causes of diabetes which means that if you're in the pre-diabetes stage, controlling

your weight can actually help prevent the problem from occurring. It manages to do this by suppressing the appetite, rendering the need to munch or graze on sweet food to a minimum. Marijuana usually produces the "munchies" instead of suppressing the appetite. Again, CBD is just a component of marijuana and thus, does not carry all of its properties.

- Diabetics also have a higher chance of suffering from infections or complications on open wounds. This is because they have a slower healing rate compared to someone without diabetes. Hence, the wounds are open for longer periods of time – increasing the chances of some bacteria penetrating through the skin. Since CBD oil has antibacterial properties, you can apply it on the skin to speed up the healing and potentially prevent the infection.

It must be noted that people with Type 2 Diabetes typically take in more medications to help with their health. Often, a person diagnosed with diabetes is also diagnosed with high blood pressure. That being the case, they may be taking as much as 3 pills in a day. If this is you, then make a point of asking your doctor about the possibility of using CBD oil together with your maintenance pills. Use of CBD oil for Type 1 Diabetes is the same as its use for Type 2 Diabetes.

Alzheimer's Disease

Remember that CBD Oil has neurocognitive properties that help with neurodegenerative diseases as already mentioned in this book. The likelihood of them helping with Alzheimer's has been proven over recent studies, showing that CBD actually helps prevent the degeneration of cognitive functions. How are you supposed to implement it for this purpose? Again, oral intake is the best – usually by placing the oil under your tongue before swallowing.

Reduce Anxiety and Depression

CBD oil has properties which connect with the neurons of the body, producing effects that primarily have something to do with a person's mood. Studies have shown that when taken by people suffering from anxiety and depression, the varied symptoms of the problems are remarkably lessened. How is this manifested?

- First, a person who takes CBD oil on a regular basis gets a better control on their mood and suffers through less palpitation or anxiety during stressful situations
- Anxious and depressed individuals also report better sleep when using CBD oil. With lack of sleep being a main contributor towards stress and anxiety, having a good night's sleep can deeply restore a person's sense of balance and wellbeing.
- CBD oil also helps relax the muscles as well as alleviate pain. It has anti-inflammatory properties which is perfect for those who have had a rough day and just want to relax before going to sleep.

In order to use CBD oil for depression and anxiety, you'll have to take CBD oil on a regular basis instead of only when you actually need it. Studies on the subject have administered CBD oil in either 400mg or 600mg dosages per day, usually through soft gels or capsules. Since you're unsure of your dosage however, it's best to start off with CBD oil use taken orally or through a vaporizer initiating a small dosage.

Stop Smoking with CBD Oil

Most of what you need to know about using CBD oil to help stop smoking has already been discussed previously in this book. As mentioned, the best way to use CBD oil for anti-smoking needs is through an e-liquid which you can load in your vaporizer tank and consume throughout the day. The beauty here is that while you may be using CBD oil primarily to stop smoking, you can also gain the various benefits that comes with its consumption. Note that if you're using CBD oil through a specialized vaporizer, you'd want to make sure that the vaporizer is being used exclusively for CBD oil.

Cooking with CBD Oil

What if you want use CBD oil merely as a supplement or to add it to your diet? The good news is that you can cook with CBD oil – but not in the straightforward sense. You can't put some CBD oil on the pan and start frying with it. So how do you incorporate CBD oil in your diet? Later on in this book, we'll provide you with CBD oil recipes.

Warning: Do NOT Diffuse CBD Oil

There are basically three ways that CBD oil can be processed to a gaseous state. There's the vaping technique, the nebulizer, and finally, a diffuser. The diffuser is the same one used for essential oils, loading the liquid into the device so as to disperse the amazing smell of the oil all over the room.

However, this is not something that can be done with CBD oil. This is because CBD oil molecules are heavier than most. Hence, a diffuser will not be able to lift up the molecules of CBD oil – which means that it will stay in the compartment. You won't be able to get the benefits of the product but simply create a more concentrated version of CBD oil.

CHAPTER EIGHT

SUCCESS STORIES AND CASE STUDIES

The internet is literally teeming with success stories and case studies with respect to CBD oil and how it helped them recover from one ailment or another. While these are definitely encouraging, keep in mind that not everything published online is factual. In this Chapter, we'll try to look through these Success Stories and present the ones with positive results backed up by Science to show you that this is not just some hype.

American Cancer Society

When it comes to cancer authority, the American Cancer Society is definitely one of the most influential associations in today's society. The official statement of the American Cancer Society is that they support the proliferation of more scientific research with respect to cannabinoids on cancer patients. This is tantamount to an admission that there is a likelihood of CBD having positive effects – just that the actual effect cannot be properly determined as of yet.

Furthermore, the society noted that many limitations imposed on the scientific community with respect to cannabinoid study. This is because as mentioned, the US Drug Enforcement Administration has maintained its classification of cannabis as a Schedule 1 Controlled Substance.

Medications Based on CBD

Another degree of acceptance of CBD in society is manifested through the introduction of certain drugs that were actually based on marijuana use. These two drugs are now approved within the United States for medical use.

- Nabilone – this is actually synthetic and leans more towards being THC than CBD. It has the same effect as THC in that it helps with nausea and preventing vomiting of cancer patients undergoing chemotherapy. This is usually a last-resort drug, taken only when other methods have not worked.
- Dronabinol – again, this is a drug that's more THC then CBD. It has been approved by the FDA or the US Food and Drug Administration for people suffering through nausea. Interestingly, the gelatin capsule is also used to help people with AIDS suffering from weight loss and lack of appetite.
- Nabiximol – is a promising spray drug that's available in Canada but still under study within the United States. The mouth spray is a combination of THC and CBD and often used to help with cancer issues, muscle spasms, and pain. It is marketed to people who have multiple sclerosis, epilepsy, and those undergoing chemotherapy treatment.

CBD Use in Treatment-Resistant Seizures

Authored by the following people: G. Pesántez-Ríos, L. Armijos-Acurio, R. Jimbo-Sotomayor, S.I. Pascual-Pascual, G. Pesántez-Cuesta, this case study shows how CBD can be used for seizures that are deemed resistant to traditional medications. Specifically, these treatment-resistant seizures are known as refractory epilepsy from which roughly 16 million people suffer from. The total number of people who suffer from epilepsy – drug resistant or otherwise – is estimated at 50 million.

The Case Study involved 15 patients which is granted, a small sample. However, this sample was studied over a period of years with CBD administered to them on a regular basis. For control purposes, the patients were first studied without CBD, finding out the extent of their seizures, the neuropsychological defects, and how the family would react to the use of CBD. In the study spanning one year, here's what they found out:

- Neurocognitive changes were impressive as 100% of these patients reported an improvement on their mood while using CBD
- The frequency of seizures also decreased by as much as 40% while in 27% of the patients, the seizures actually disappeared completely!
- The study also revealed that 60% of the patients were able to control their seizures 50% of the time

Are there any drawbacks? Unfortunately, the use of CBD also increased sleepiness in many of the patients.

CBD and High Blood Pressure Reduction

One of the most prevalent health issues today, high blood pressure is often termed as the silent killer. In this study, it was shown that CBD can actually help with high blood pressure. More specifically, a study by Khalid A. Jadoon, Garry D. Tan, and Saoirse E. O'Sullivan show that it reduces the resting systolic blood pressure through the introduction of 600mg CBD on healthy volunteers.

The results were compared to a placebo group for control purposes and the result was conclusive. This means that while diet and exercise can help with high blood pressure, adding CBD to the array of possible high blood pressure treatments is a distinct possibility.

It should also be noted that lowering blood pressure must also be considered as a side effect when taken by people who are using CBD for entirely different reasons. For example, people with hypotension using CBD for pain relief should consider the possibility that the CBD will negatively impact their already low blood pressure.

CBD and Schizophrenia

This section features research by: Osborne AL, Solowij N, Weston-Green K; Illawarra Health and Medical Research Institute of the University of Wollongong

It's been mentioned often enough that CBD can help with psychotic disorders which includes schizophrenia. In this case study involving years of research, the proponents have noted the clear connection between CBD and schizophrenia. To put it into simple terms – it has been found that CBD can be an alternative to prescription drugs used to treat schizophrenia. In fact, it has the promise of being a healthier and safer alternative compared to traditional drugs that come with extreme side effects.

This conclusion was arrived at after studying articles over the past 26 years involving schizophrenia and CBD use. Accordingly, the introduction of CBD in the system helps improve cognitive abilities of patients and delays cognitive impairment. Interestingly enough, the anti-psychotic characteristic of CBD is not limited to

Schizophrenia but also includes Alzheimer 's disease, Epilepsy, and other neuro-inflammatory conditions.

Seizures in Children with CBD

Authors are: Orrin Devinsky, M.D., J. Helen Cross, Ph.D., F.R.C.P.C.H., Linda Laux, M.D., Eric Marsh, M.D., Ian Miller, M.D., Rima Nabbout, M.D., Ingrid E. Scheffer, M.B., B.S., Ph.D., Elizabeth A. Thiele, M.D., Ph.D., and Stephen Wright, M.D.; Cannabidiol in Dravet Syndrome Study Group

This is definitely one of the most important studies in CBD today considering the prevalence of seizures in children and the difficulty of finding a safe drug to help manage their condition. This case study is focused on patients with Dravet Syndrome which is a rare neurological disorder which becomes evident as early as one year old. Due to the youth of the patients, it can be terribly difficult to find the right dosage for the patient. This study was conducted over 120 children and young adults diagnosed with the condition. The double blind study is also placebo controlled to ensure success.

The study covered a 14-week period whereby the patients were orally administered with CBD on the basis of their weight and taking into consideration their regular dosage if given traditional medicine. This was the result.

- **CBD-treated convulsive seizures decreased from 12.4 to 5.9 percent**
- The placebo group only decreased by 0.8 percent
- Wonderfully, **5% of patients who were given CBD became** *seizure free*, compared with none in the placebo group.

The drawback is that there are side effects, particularly experienced by those in the CBD group with respect to vomiting and fever.

CHAPTER NINE

SIMPLE CBD OIL RECIPES

As already mentioned, you can't be expected to cook with CBD Oil through traditional means. You can't put it in a pan and expect to fry food with it. However, CBD Oil is much like olive oil – you can add it in any recipe any it just improves the taste or sometimes, doesn't change the taste at all. Here are some recipes you can try out:

Chocolate Chip Cookies with CBD

- 1 cup softened butter
- 2 tsp. vanilla extract
- 3 cups of flour
- 1 tsp. baking soda
- 1 cup white sugar
- 2 tsp. hot water
- 1 cup brown sugar
- 2 eggs
- ½ tsp. salt

- 0.5 oz. unflavored CBD oil

- 2 cups semisweet chocolate chips

Preheat your oven to 350 degrees Fahrenheit.

Mix all the wet ingredients thoroughly until you get a cream like consistency.

Don't include the eggs yet though. Beat them in a separate bowl and add the vanilla.

Add flour to the mix and combine them thoroughly. Combine the baking soda with hot water so that it thoroughly dissolves before adding in the salt.

Bring in the chocolate chips. When done, layer them all out on the baking sheet, making sure there's around 2 inches of space between each dollop. Bake for 10 minutes.

Guacamole Dip with CBD

- 1 tsp. CBD oil

- 1 tsp. salt

- 1 tsp. minced garlic

- ½ cup diced onion

- 3 tbs. chopped cilantro

- 3 avocados

- 1 lime

- 2 diced tomatoes

Mash up the avocados. Put in the lime juice, salt, and CBD oil.

Once done, put the other vegetables and taste your end result. Add more salt, pepper, and other seasonings depending on your personal preferences.

CBD Peppermint Chocolate Cups

- 3/4 cup Rawmio Essentials mint chocolate, or Veggimins CBD dark chocolate chopped or vegan dark chocolate chip

- 1/4 cup Raw Guru cacao butter (2 oz)

- 2 Tbsp raw cashew butter

- 1/4 cup Dastony coconut butter

- 1 tsp pure vanilla extract

- 2 Tbsp maple syrup

- 1/8 tsp sea salt

- 1/4 tsp matcha powder or spinach powder

Start by melting the dark chocolate until it is completely smooth. Place some of this dark chocolate in peanut butter cup molds. Put them in the freezer until they're hard. This is where the fun begins.

Grab the cacao butter, cashew butter, maple syrup, vanilla, and sea salt. Whisk until cream and smooth. When they're well blended, you can add the CBD oil and the matcha powder.

Take the chocolate cups out of the fridge and pour your white chocolate on top. Place back in the freezer and take them out again when you want to eat them!

Pumpkin Spice Latte Loaf

- 1 Tbsp Fire Cider
- 1 tsp baking soda
- 4 eggs
- 1 cup pure pumpkin puree
- 1/2 cup Otto's Cassava Flour
- 1 Tbsp Biovelle CBD coconut oil
- 1/4 cup coconut butter
- 1 tsp espresso powder
- 1 tsp pumpkin pie spice

Combine Fire Cider and baking soda into a bowl. Put in the eggs and start using an electric mixer to get that beautiful blend.

Add in all the other ingredients except the CBD coconut oil and the coconut butter since you'll be using those for the icing.

Mix well until you're ready to pour them into the loaf pan. Baking time should be around 30 minutes at 350 degrees Fahrenheit. When done, take them out and put them in the fridge while you make the icing.

The icing is simple enough. Just melt the CBD coconut oil and coconut butter together. When properly melted, pour them over the loaf. If you managed to cool down the load by putting it in the fridge, then the icing will harden immediately. Serve and done!

CBD Infused Butter CBD

- 2 cups butter

- 20 ML CBD oil

- 1 cup water

Just chop the butter into small pieces and combine them all into one pot. Heat them in a low setting for 2 solid hours, making sure to stir consistently to avid lumps. Once the mixture cools a little, pour it into a container that you'll be using as a mold. Once done, you can put it in the fridge and use it just like real butter. The beauty of this is that this makes it very easy to include CBD in your day to day life as you use the butter in numerous recipes.

CBD Gummies

- 1 cup tart cherry juice

- 1/4 cup gelatin powder

- 2 T raw honey

- CBD oil

Start by putting the juice into a saucepan and apply medium heat. Pour in the gelatin but do so slowly, mixing all the while.

After a thorough mix, add the honey, keeping the heat low all the while. Just keep stirring until the gelation has fully dissolved.

When done, take it out of the fire and pour in your CBD oil. Mix a little bit more before putting them in your molds. It should harden completely when in the fridge for around 2 hours. From there, you can take them out of the mold and store them in an airtight container, lasting for up to 2 weeks.

These gummies are ideal for those who need a good night's sleep. Just take one or two an hour before you're ready to go to bed.

CBD Bliss Balls

- ¾ cup macadamia nuts (I used roasted and salted, but raw works too)
- 1 tablespoon coconut oil, melted
- ⅓ cup unsweetened shredded coconut
- ½ teaspoon ground cinnamon
- 1 teaspoon pure vanilla extract
- 1 tablespoon (120 mg) CBD-infused MCT oil
- ⅓ cup almond flour
- 2 tablespoons cacao nibs

Put the macadamia nuts in a blender and grind them until you get a pasty cream.

Pour in the CBD oil and the melted coconut oil. Blend them some more until you get a thick consistency – a lot like butter.

Once done, put them in a large bowl and pour the almond flour, shredded coconut, vanilla, and ground cinnamon. Mix them all together thoroughly. The end result would be a cookie dough texture. Add some salt or sugar as needed by tasting the dough.

Fold the cacao nibs and scoop some of the dough between your palms. Roll them together until you're sure that the balls are tight. This should produce around 10 balls in all.

Refrigerate them afterwards and eat them as you wish! They should last for 1 month if kept in the freezer.

Additional Tips for Cooking with CBD

When cooking with CBD you can add the oil in the mix and just follow the traditional recipe you have. Feel free to explore and experiment with your CBD recipes to see which one tastes best for you. Note though that there are several rules to follow when cooking with CBD oil.

- Make sure the oil is still good or that it has been properly stored and therefore can be added to food without any adverse effects. Smell the oil first and make a judgment call as to its smell. To prolong your CBD oil, make sure to store it in a cool and dry place away from direct sunlight.
- Make sure to stir the oil thoroughly into the mixture to prevent coagulation.
- Try not to go overboard with the amount of CBD you're using. There's no rule of thumb as to how much CBD oil you should add in a recipe but in the interest of safety, try not to go beyond 600mg for each batch.
- You can also try adding CBD oil to your shakes or juices to have that added boost. You won't feel a thing with respect to taste or texture – but you'll be glad to know that there's an added ingredient there that helps with your overall health.

CHAPTER TEN

FREQUENTLY ASKED QUESTIONS

Now that we're wrapping up this book on CBD Hemp Oil, we'll try to tackle some of the most common questions asked by people when taking the product. Read on and find out some of the most commonly asked questions in the industry:

Will CBD Hemp Oil make me fail a drug test?

No. Unless you're taking a THC-rich CBD oil, then you should be fine when it comes to drug tests. This is because drugs tests look for a specific cannabinoid which is THC – the intoxicating compound that forms part of marijuana. CBD is a whole kettle of fish and thus, will not register when it comes to drug tests. Since THC in CBD Oil is usually less than 0.3 percent, then traditional tests would not register the THC amount.

Can I use CBD as a supplement?

Yes – even if you don't have health problems, you can still use CBD oil as a possible source of supplement for your day to day needs. There's nothing wrong with adding it to your health routine – provided that the CBD oil is legal in your area. Note though that if you have pre-existing health conditions, you'll have to make sure that there's a go signal from your physician to take the supplement.

Can I Extract CBD Myself?

This one is a fairly interesting question and there's really no straightforward answer. Simply put, you can extract CBD Oil yourself – but it's usually not advisable. Also note that in order to extract CBD oil, you'll need access to cannabis or hemp – and this is not possible if cannabis is considered illegal in your area. If not however, you can try some of the processes here that are ideal for home-extractions.

- Use of ethanol – there's really no need for you to have an advance degree in science in order to extract CBD oil through the use of ethanol. The beauty of this technique is that the resulting taste of the oil is as pure and as clean as possible. The drawback is that it destroys the waxy substance of the cannabis which is often considered as beneficial to the overall health of a person. Here's how to do this:

  o Take the weed and place it in a bowl. Grab some alcohol and pour it in the bowl. Stir for 6 to 10 minutes using a wooden spoon. It helps if the weed has been chopped or mashed a little bit so that the juices can flow out of it faster.

  o Once you're done, place the weed out of the bowl and place it in a bag or a clean cloth. Start squeezing the cloth to extract as much resin as possible from the weed.

  o Repeat the process for as long as you can get a bit of liquid or oil from the weed. The volume of your results would primarily depend on how hard you squeeze the weed product.

o At this point, you've got a combination of oil and alcohol in the squeezed bowl. The goal now is to remove the ethanol by heating it up.

o Place the resulting liquid in a pan and turn on the fire, making sure it's low and steady. Wait until the bubbles start to appear and the alcohol starts to evaporate. When all the alcohol has evaporated, you can turn off the flame completely and just mix the oil.

o Place the oil in a storage bottle. Keep the lid tight because CBD oil can go bad when not properly sealed, thereby reducing its effectiveness.

o You'll note that this very straightforward approach does not take into account the possibility that THC is also included in the squeezed oil. This is why individuals are advised to use only cannabis plants that have a low concentration of THC. This way, you can be sure that the result is also low in THC.

- Olive Oil – the use of olive oil is perhaps the easiest way to extract CBD from marijuana. Again, you'll need to use cannabis that's already high in CBD with low THC content.

    o Start by exposing the weed through a process called decarboxylation. This is when you bake the weed at 220 degrees Fahrenheit for 90 minutes.

    o Once you're done baking, you can now grind the weed, choosing the parts you actually want to use for your oil. As already mentioned, a whole plant extraction is usually better because this means you'll be getting nutrients from all parts of the plant.

o Place the weed inside a mason jar and pour the oil of your choice. In this tutorial, we're using olive oil but you can also use coconut oil.

o Saturate the weed in coconut oil so that it binds to every part of the cannabis plant.

o The next step is to grab a pan and place some water inside it. Take a towel and put it on the bottom of the pan. Grab your mason jar and secure the lid in place.

o Put the Mason jar in the pan and turn on the oven. Allow the water to reach a boiling point but not too much. You want the boil to be low, long, and steady at just 200 degrees. A thermometer will be very useful here because if the heat is too much, you can burn the oil. If too low, then you're not going to extract the oil you want.

o Leave it there for about 3 hours – yes, it takes that long to process the CBD oil! You'll have to check every now and again to make sure there's still water in the pot. Once you've finished the 3 hour requirement, you can turn off the fire and leave the Mason jar there for another 3 hours. Heat again for 3 hours, turn off the heat, and then leave it there overnight

o Strain the CBD oil using a clean cloth or a cheese cloth for a more precise squeeze. Place the oil inside a tight container and keep it in a cool and dry place. Note that the concentration of the CBD oil would depend on the amount of coconut or olive oil you use. With more olive oil, the less the concentration would be.

Other extraction methods such as the use of carbon dioxide – as previously mentioned in this book – are available, but not ideal. In the first place, you'll need sophisticated equipment in order to make the extraction. There's also the question of whether you can actually separate the CBD oil from the THC or the intoxicating compound of the cannabis plant.

How long before I see results?

The length of time it takes before you see results depends largely on the method of ingestion you use. Vaping or smoking CBD is probably the quickest but not exactly ideal if you want to benefit from the purest version of the product. CBD than can be smoked usually comes with thinning agents with messes up with the dosage. The best ways therefore would be through oral ingestion – either through tincture or through capsules. In both methods, you can expect results in a matter of hours – the same way as traditional medication. The benefits are instantaneous and should give you the relief you need quickly enough.

CONCLUSION

To wrap it up, CBD Oil is one of the most promising health products in the market today. It's so popular that some people term it as a super food because of the wide and varied benefits it allegedly provides its users.

While most of these claims are still unconfirmed, they are the subject of ongoing studies that veer towards positive results. The fact that you're reading this book means that you're open to the possibility of CBD Oil being a common element in the health care of the future.

Due to the fact that there's still little regulation as to CBD, your choice of using it is completely up to you. Hopefully, this book was able to guide you in making your decision with respect to CBD use, how to use it, and how to best approach the product as a natural medicine for your many ailments.

It is greatly encouraged that as more information about CBD enters the market, you also update your sources and find out the conclusions arrived at by top scientists in the niche.

www.ingramcontent.com/pod-product-compliance
Lightning Source LLC
Chambersburg PA
CBHW020616220526
45463CB00006B/2599